NO KALE REQUIRED!

Healthy Eating Ideas
for the Rest of Us!

NANCY OGLESBY

dedication

This book is dedicated to my husband Jim. His life and death transformed me into the person I am today. I am forever grateful for his love.

No Kale Required
Healthy Eating Ideas for the Rest of Us

Cover/Interior Design: NJO Consulting
Published by: HealthWorksKC LLC

Copyright © 2016 Nancy Oglesby

ISBN-10: 0-9985141-1-X

ISBN-13: 978-0-9985141-1-6

acknowledgements

I want to acknowledge people who helped me learn about healthy living starting with my sister, Pat Douglas. I've always looked up to Pat and it was her early adventures with "Let's Eat Well to Keep Fit" by Adelle Davis that brought healthy living into my awareness. As a James Scholar to the University of Illinois, and self-professed grammar geek, she was the perfect choice to be my copy editor. I am grateful that she agreed!

It was my son Scott's lifestyle change that spurred my own. (He's now my racquetball partner and exhibits an amazing level of patience!)

Joshua Rosenthal, Founder of the Institute for Integrative Nutrition in New York City developed a program that not only educates but inspires as well. Choosing to attend was a great decision.

I'd also like to thank Marcie for being my accountability partner, Teresa, Mary Ann, Cyndi, Chris, Mary, Bob, Jana, Jan, Brian and Julie for their input, and encouragement along the way. A big thanks to Mike Deathe whose informative presentation on writing a book was the fuel thrown on the No Kale Required fire. And to my first client, Becky for trusting me then, and now. She is one of many clients and students I've learned from since this journey began.

If I've forgotten anyone they're sure to forgive me because they're used to the effects of ADHD, my super power. ☺ It most definitely takes a village!

I would be remiss if I didn't express gratitude for the pups that sat silently (actually, they cuddled on their bed) as I worked to get this finished. They were good pooches! Oh yeah ... and the cat.

about the author

Nancy is a cat with many lives! Her motto? Never get bored! She's been a Graphic Designer at a Chicagoland studio, Special Projects Manager at G.D. Searle Pharmaceuticals, Ground Operations Manager at FedEx Express and a Marketing Consultant.

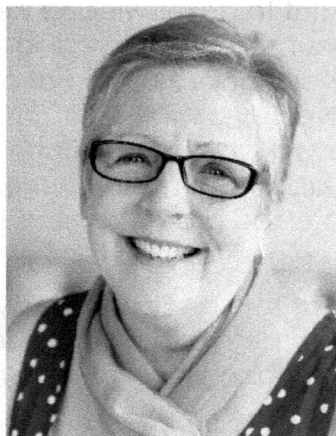

In 2009 she found herself without health insurance for the first time ever! Instead of being completely stressed, Nancy decided to get healthy. That was when she found her passion: healthy food, nutrition and natural wellness, plus the desire to guide and support others on their journey to healthy living.

As a 2011 graduate of the Institute for Integrative Nutrition, her passion is to make healthy lifestyle changes accessible to everyone. Education is the key. She teaches classes, coaches, designs wellness programs, does lunch & learns for small businesses and organizations and writes feature articles ... all of which keep boredom at bay!

table of contents

I invite you to think of each idea as a stepping stone on your journey. No two paths are alike so for me to design the path would likely lead to people falling by the wayside, but when you lay the stones out in your own unique combination, you'll be on your way to success!

Each idea presented here can change your health for the better, and I've included practical ways to help you make them work. Some ideas are easier than others, but I think I've given you some great tools to get started.

Let's get healthy!

"Life isn't about finding yourself. Life's about creating yourself." ~ George Bernard Shaw

introduction

So, you want to change your lifestyle from unhealthy to healthy, but every time you try you do great for a while and then KA-BAM! you're back to your old habits. What the heck? This was the way my life went forever—until I figured out that if I could make one simple change at a time, rather than changing everything, those simple changes would add up to one seriously BIG change over time!

This series will take you through a new way of thinking about lifestyle changes, giving you the opportunity to wade into the ocean instead of diving in headfirst! It's designed to be flexible and gives you complete control. For example:

Let's say that your physician wants you to lose 25lbs. by eating right and exercising more. Instead of rushing to the grocery store to buy hundreds of dollars of healthy food, then dashing to sign up at the gym, take some time to sit down and think about how best to accomplish this.

Are you a single mom of two kids, working full time? Chances are good that by Day 3 those hundreds of dollars of healthy food will go to waste because you won't actually be fixing them, and forget getting to the gym every day. Day 2 concludes with your daughter's cheerleading competition that was supposed to end at 6:15 but went much longer. You still have to get home, fix dinner, help with homework and finish that spreadsheet that you brought home from the office because you need it for a 7AM meeting. Whew! There goes the idea of actually getting in any gym time.

So, without a reality check, your plans will most likely fail. Some days are nearly impossible to get through without having to focus on new food, new exercise, new this and new that. It will depend on your goals, but you'll need to determine what you want to focus on first.

I'm starting out with *No Kale Required: Healthy Eating Ideas for the Rest of Us* because food is what builds our cells, and our cells are constantly regenerating. This means that you have the choice to build healthy cells or junk food cells.

Read through the choices and pick one to begin with. I've written several sections so that you've got all kinds of changes to choose from. But let's be honest, a few of these are pretty big and will take more time to achieve than others. It might even take more than a year for you to be comfortable with them. On the bright side, there are several that are super simple, so while you're working on a big one you can be adding in some of the smaller ones.

Keeping a record of your changes is a great motivator! You can track your progress using the tracking sheets at the back of the book, or use any method of tracking that works for you.

Let's go!

eat whole foods

Synergy. That's the big deal. Did you know that an apple has over 400 compounds in it? 400! Scientists have identified over 10,000 compounds in fruits and vegetables, but the scientists over at ABC Multivitamin Corporation (I sure hope there's not an actual company by that name!) have decided on 32 or 43 or 12 as the magic number of nutrients that will work for you. Next, they create synthetics or isolate naturals and pack them into a pill and call it good. Apparently, all it takes is a handful of isolated nutrients to support your system's nutritional needs.

The trouble is that your body didn't get the memo and doesn't quite know what to do with those isolated nutrients when they aren't ingested with the other hundreds and thousands of naturally-occurring compounds found in fruits and vegetables. Scientists are beginning to catch up with what Mother Nature already knew: we are a part of the ecosystem we live in and as such, we are designed to work best with the whole orange rather than just the Vitamin C, with the whole carrot, not the isolated Vitamin A. Do yourself a favor and stick with whole foods.

According to Nutrition Source[i], a publication of the Harvard School of Public Health, results of the most effective type of studies (randomized, placebo-controlled trials) haven't supported taking single antioxidants (vitamin C, E and/or vitamin A, among others). Results tend to be negative rather than positive in their use in the prevention of cancer, heart disease and other chronic conditions.

As I've discussed with students and clients, the reductionist thinking that has been leading the charge in nutritional science for decades is coming under attack for ignoring nature's delivery systems ... the foods themselves. Taking beta-carotene out of the carrot or sweet potato doesn't work as well, if at all, and in some cases is harmful.

Each whole food has its own unique system of delivery and science is showing that the body often doesn't know what to do with nutrients when they're in a form other than that which nature provided. So, eat whole, brown rice, quinoa, oats, whole wheat, barley, real eggs and lean meat, beans, legumes, greens and every fruit and veggie you can think of!

We don't have a vitamin deficiency in this country. Just walk into any grocery or drug store and you'll see an entire aisle devoted to them. What we have is a whole food deficiency that has led us to being one of the unhealthiest nations in the world! It's time to take back your health!

eat an apple

There are tons of phytonutrients including resveratrol, flavonoids, carotenoids ... you don't really want to know all of this do you? So, here's what you need to know: apples are really good for you. Research tells us the old saying "an apple a day keeps the doctor away," has the ring of truth to it.

The beauty of apples is that there's an apple for everyone! Do you like tart? Try a Granny Smith or Pink Lady. Are you looking for something sweeter? Gala and Fuji come to mind.

And, you can eat them how you choose, whole or sliced, room temperature or ice cold, with peanut butter or without. Your choice!

Here are just a few of the benefits of adding apples into your diet:

- Reduction in the risk of cancer and dementia
- Supports regular elimination (diarrhea or constipation)
- Helps to control your weight and can reduce the risk of Type 2 Diabetes
- In a study in the UK researchers found that an apple a day was as effective as statins in the prevention of cardiovascular deaths[ii].

According to the website, The World's Healthiest Foods (one of my favorites), it's not just the pectin in apples that's responsible for the apple's ability to reduce blood fat; it's the synergy that occurs between the pectin and all of the other phytonutrients[iii]. So, eat an apple. It's that simple!

be good to your gut

Do you like sauerkraut? How about sour pickles or red cabbage? Have you tried yogurt, kimchi, kombucha or kefir? Adding in fermented foods to your daily regimen can improve your gut health drastically. In my kitchen it's an absolute staple.

If you do any research into fermented foods and probiotics you'll learn that there are many different types of bacteria, plus a few other little buggers (viruses, fungi) living in and on our bodies. There are over 100 trillion microbes in the gut alone, more microbes than human body cells[iv].

These dudes are important! The trouble is that we routinely kill them off when we use antimicrobial soaps, hand sanitizers and cleaners that remove them from our personal environment. It doesn't help that antibiotics are overprescribed and fed to the animals that end up on our plates.

Our microbiome (the name for all of those little critters as a whole) is being researched in conjunction with inflammatory bowel disease, obesity, allergic and autoimmune diseases and several neuropsychiatric issues such as autism, schizophrenia, chronic fatigue, obsessive compulsive and mood disorders, anorexia, and attention deficit disorder. It is becoming increasingly clear just how important our microbiome is to our ability to resist chronic disease.

The least expensive way to go about adding in these

foods is to make them yourself. There are Facebook groups dedicated to fermenting, along with the website Cultured Food Life where you can get a beginner's guide for free.

When you add in fermented foods make sure to try a variety of products. There are more fermented foods to choose from than ever before. Most stores like Whole Foods, Trader Joe's, Natural Grocers and Sprouts have them available. I love, love, love Trader Joe's spicy fermented cauliflower.

Things that negatively impact your microbiome include a diet of processed foods and too much sugar, overuse of antibiotics by individuals as well as by agriculture, and caesarian births that eliminate the 'seeding' that occurs as a newborn travels through the vaginal canal[v.]

Recognizing the importance of this issue, the Mayo Clinic has a *Clinician's Primer on the Role of the Microbiome in Human Health and Disease*, designed specifically to educate physicians on the emerging science surrounding the connection between the microbiome and a person's health.

If you'd like to eat a diet that supports your microbiome, visit www.drweil.com and click on the Anti-Inflammatory Diet Pyramid.

eat large at lunch

Are you having trouble losing weight despite your efforts? Why not try what researchers have found successful? Eat the bulk of your calories earlier in the day.

When I was in my twenties I worked as a graphic designer at a residential community for adults with Downs Syndrome. The community included a pet store, small petting zoo, silk screen shop, bakery and restaurant where residents worked (and played) every day.

The restaurant had the best homemade food EVER and I had the luxury of eating there every day at almost no cost. (I think it was fifty cents!) Each day I would fill my plate with deliciousness. The day's meal might include meatloaf, mashed potatoes and gravy, a vegetable, a lovely green salad, apple pie and a glass of lemonade. I didn't count calories and there was no paying attention to gluten, dairy or meat, after all, it was the 70's!

Did I gain weight? Nope, I lost weight! Why? Because I was totally satisfied, ate a small dinner and very rarely snacked in the evening. I'm not saying this was a healthy diet for me, with my genetics I shouldn't be regularly indulging in meat, sweets and mashed potatoes, but what I learned is that eating a large lunch can change your cravings the rest of the day—and that's not the only benefit.

By eating your largest meal early, you're giving your body the opportunity to use that food for fuel rather than storing it. Americans tend to sit after dinner, watching television or reading, but after lunch we're still mobile. Having your largest meal before 3PM is a great way to allow your body to use the food as fuel rather than to store it as it is likely to do when eaten later in the evening.

What's the rule of thumb you might use if you choose this habit? Eat a good breakfast, a larger lunch and a small dinner with no snacking in the evening hours. If your weight loss calorie count is 1400 calories, aim for a 350 calorie breakfast, 700 calorie lunch and 350 calories at dinner.

reduce red meat

In the Introduction I mentioned that some challenges might take longer than a month. This is one of them, but a lot of good things happen when you reduce your consumption of red meat. Typically, you will see a reduction in LDL (the bad cholesterol), you'll most likely lose weight, and you will definitely be lowering your risk of heart disease, stroke and cancer.

Just what meats will you be reducing? Bologna, hot dogs, packaged ham, deli beef, hamburgers, roast beef, barbeque ribs, pork, brisket, pot roast, sausage or pepperoni pizza, bacon, sausage gravy ... you get the idea? You hate me, right?

Remember, I only said to *reduce* your consumption. By far the worst culprit is processed meat, so if you want to start on your health journey super slow, just cut out deli meats to begin. There are some very tasty alternatives. Here are just a few of them:

- Uncured bologna and hot dogs made from chicken, turkey or tofu (don't shudder, it's not nice!)
- Joe's Kansas City has fabulous barbeque chicken sandwiches—check out what's available in your area.
- Ask the pizza place to go easy on the toppings
- Make your biscuits and gravy at home with uncured turkey sausage
- Make yourself a sliced chicken or turkey sandwich.

Instead of using deli meats, buy a rotisserie chicken, slice it up and you'll have enough for dinner and sandwiches as well. (If you're really adventurous, toss the carcass in some water, add an onion, parsley, salt, pepper, garlic, and carrots, cook for several hours, strain, and you've got homemade chicken broth. Pick out any meat that's left and add it back into the broth and you've got a great base for chicken soup. Now all you need are a few veggies and rice or noodles for another meal!)

Alternate chicken sandwiches with tuna salad or peanut butter and jelly to keep things interesting. Adding in grilled cod in a delicious fish taco is just one more way to diversify your menu. You can also check the internet for more ideas for healthy alternatives.

When it's time for red meat, make it worth it: bacon on Sunday mornings or a burger at your favorite burger joint.

Your heart will love you!

milk is for baby cows

My story: In my fifties, I decided to give up red meat and dairy for two reasons: first, to reduce my cholesterol, second for animal rights reasons. It was harder to police agricultural practices than it was to just quit consuming the product.

What happened as a result was that my arthritis was diminished, but even more surprisingly, my asthma attacks went away completely and my sensitivities to fragrances and chemicals lessened significantly. I no longer started sneezing or wheezing when I was around someone with perfume or aftershave on, and I could go out in my yard, or open my windows when my neighbors were drying their clothes with dryer sheets. This was almost a normal life!

Twenty years before that I decided to see if there was a medical reason that caused my lifelong difficulty with breathing through my nose. I was diagnosed with chronic rhinitis and told to inhale salt water daily. It didn't do much and was an annoying process so I quit doing it almost as soon as I started. Imagine my surprise after I quit eating cheese and ice cream when I realized I could breathe through my nose for the first time in my life!

On my experience alone I can recommend that people eliminate dairy from their diets, but you don't have to rely on my word alone. Food journalist Mark Bittman wrote a fabulous piece on dairy (July 7, 2012) and a few weeks later followed it up with another after receiving so many comments and emails. As he wrote in the New York Times on July 24th, 2012:

"Not surprisingly, experiences like mine with dairy, outlined in my column of two weeks ago, are more common than unusual, at least according to the roughly 1,300 comments and e-mails we received since then. In them, people outlined their experiences with dairy and health problems as varied as heartburn, migraines, irritable bowel syndrome, colitis, eczema, acne, hives, asthma ("When I gave up dairy, my asthma went away completely"), gall bladder issues, body aches, ear infections, colic, "seasonal allergies," rhinitis, chronic sinus infections and more. (One writer mentioned an absence of canker sores after cutting dairy; I realized I hadn't had a canker sore — which I've gotten an average of once a month my whole life — in four months. Something else to think about.)[vi]"

As Mr. Bittman pointed out in his original article, his esophageal reflux (GERD) went away completely when he eliminated dairy[vii]. Turns out his canker sores and asthma are gone as well. I lost my asthma too ... What might change in your health with this one, simple change?

There are great alternatives to milk, including nut, hemp, flax, soy, and rice milks. For drinking you'll probably prefer vanilla. I've found that unsweetened almond or coconut milk can be used in just about any cream sauce and even for biscuits and gravy! (Don't forget to use uncured turkey sausage.)

Cheese alternatives were a little trickier until Field Roast came out with their latest product, Chao alternative cheese. It comes in a few different flavors, but the original is my favorite. Fast on their heels was Follow Your Heart® with an American, Provolone, Garden Herb and Mozzarella cheese alternative that is also delicious. Both taste good by the slice and they melt beautifully for grilled cheese sandwiches!

You can Google 'Mark Bittman Dairy' and you'll get links to both articles. Great information!

add in some lemons

Making healthy lemonade will balance your electrolytes and quench your thirst, just go easy on the sweeteners. Using a combination of raw honey and stevia will sweeten your beverage without ruining your health.

Hot Lemonade is, hands down, my favorite little, maybe-there's-a-cold-coming-on beverage: fresh squeezed lemon, local raw honey and a sprig of rosemary. So good for you it's crazy—and so easy!

Lemons are high in vitamin C and loaded with other antioxidants which help to prevent oxidation, more commonly known as the damage caused by free radicals. Lemons have long been recognized for their immune-boosting, anti-inflammatory properties.

I love it when historical remedies are scientifically proven! Hot lemonade, whether you drink it as lemonade, add tea or make it a hot toddy by adding whiskey, has its benefits!

read labels

Don't let the food companies fool you with their pictures of fresh fruit on the front of the box, or their BIG statements such as 0 TRANS FATS. Learn to read the labels. You don't have to be able to pronounce the chemicals you'll find there, just look for things you recognize, or that you think should be in it.

The ingredients on any food are listed in descending order of the amount that's in the recipe. For instance, if sugar is listed first, that's the ingredient there's the most of in that cereal, soup or sauce mix. The ingredients on all food labels start with what there's the most of and finish with what there's the least of in that package.

It's also helpful to know a little trick that manufacturers use to fool us into thinking there's less sugar in a product. They use several different forms of sugar, listing each one separately, so that they fall further down in that descending-order ingredient list. The many names of sugar: sugar, cane sugar, honey, molasses, glucose, dextrose, high-fructose corn syrup, rice syrup, corn syrup, barley malt syrup, sorghum syrup, maltodextrin—the list is endless, and when they break it up into pieces, it doesn't look as bad to you, the consumer.

Typically, breakfast cereals with beautiful pictures of blueberries on the package have no blueberries listed on the ingredient list. What I've seen is 'blueberry flavored' or 'blueberry flavored bits' followed by a lot of chemicals in parenthesis. Occasionally, there's an actual blueberry listed, but it is often far down in the list and remember, the further down in the list, the less there is in the package.

Don't believe the marketing images of cozy kitchens and chefs coming up with delicious recipes. Become a label sleuth and read what's actually in the food you buy. There are some popular packaged lunches that have 60+ ingredients in a package less than four-ounces, and sugar is the first thing listed. Another snack item that flies off the shelf has about 115 ingredients. That's not food, that's a science experiment!

lose the trans fats

Zero trans fats is a big draw on packaging but isn't always true. The FDA allows less than half a gram (.5g) per serving to go unstated, but if you learn to read labels, you won't be fooled again. Any ingredient list that lists 'partially hydrogenated oil' means there are trans fats in the product.

If you buy cookies or chips that's got 'Zero trans fats' on the packaging, but the label has partially hydrogenated vegetable oil in the ingredient list, you are ingesting trans fats. The FDA has determined that trans fats are no longer considered 'generally safe' and they will be completely removed from our food supply by 2018. FDA's Acting Commissioner Stephen Ostroff, M.D. reports that "This action is expected to reduce coronary heart disease and prevent thousands of fatal heart attacks every year[viii]."

Why are trans fats so bad? According to the American Heart Association, trans fats raise your bad (LDL) cholesterol levels and lower your good (HDL) cholesterol levels. Eating trans fats increases your risk of developing heart disease, stroke and is associated with a higher risk of developing type 2 diabetes[ix].

Partially hydrogenated oil is found in a lot of different foods, including cookies, crackers and cakes, frozen and refrigerated dough products, any variety of chips, microwave popcorn, French fries, fried chicken, doughnuts, non-dairy creamers, and margarine.

People rarely use one serving of coffee creamer (just one tablespoon) or eat one ounce of chips ... Americans are typically getting far more trans fats than they might think.

Is there is a product you love that has partially hydrogenated oils in it? Write the company and let them know you would love to continue to be a customer, but you just can't put your heart health at risk.

get sneaky

Do you, or does someone in your family, totally resist eating veggies? If so, you need to get a little sneaky. You can hide greens in just about anything from spaghetti sauce to vegetable soup.

Try pureeing spinach, carrots or kale into your spaghetti sauce. Other than a little darker in color, no one will notice. And, with the addition of carrots you can eliminate any sugar you might add to your sauce to tame the acidity.

There are several recipes on the web for avocado chocolate pudding and they are truly delicious, easy to make, and so much more nutritious than boxed mixes or prepackaged!

If you like vegetable soup with the standard green beans, corn, carrots and peas, puree some greens (spinach, cabbage or kale) with some of the broth and add back in. The flavor is fabulous and you won't even know they're there.

Get creative and find ways to sneak those veggies in!

so delicious strawberries

Do you love strawberries? Fresh or frozen, strawberries are my favorite. Sometimes I mix them together with blueberries for a serious jolt of antioxidants, but I missed my whipped cream and I wanted to find something that was a healthier substitute.

Enter So Delicious® French Vanilla Creamer. This little treat is the perfect addition to my berries! You have to be very careful to only use a small amount since it has 25 calories and 4g of sugar per tablespoon. I use two tablespoons (and I measure every time) for 1½ cups of berries. It's not a lot, but just enough to add a little sweetness and creaminess without doing too much damage.

This is one of those things that makes me happy when I'm craving something sweet. I hope you like it!

pbj ... it's not just for kids

Nut butters are a fabulous alternative to processed meats at lunchtime. Whether you use peanut, almond or another nut butter, you are adding in heart-healthy fats, fiber and protein. A nice, dense whole grain bread topped with fresh fruit or 100% fruit spreads is a tasty and satisfying meal.

Some options include:

- peanut butter, thinly sliced granny smith apples
- peanut butter, 100% strawberry fruit spread
- peanut butter, thinly sliced dill pickles (you'll have to trust me on this!)
- almond butter, whole cranberry sauce
- almond butter, smashed bananas

I like to cut my sandwich in triangles, sit on a high wall, kick my feet back and forth and feel like a kid again. They taste almost as good even if you're stuck at your desk.

freeze everything

Well, maybe not everything, but most things. I love cherries in season, but the season is short and I can eat only so many cherries before they're gone for another year, so I freeze them, pits and all—yep! Just about any fruit or veggie can be frozen for future use. Some taste great when you eat them frozen, others I thaw and eat (think strawberries and blueberries from So Delicious Strawberries) and still others I use in smoothies, sangria, soups and stews.

There's often a banana that's about to go bad or oranges that you can't possibly eat in time. Or you can't take advantage of the sale on grapes because there's no way you can use them soon enough. Maybe you bought that bag of kale with good intentions, but the intentions didn't follow you home from the store.

How many times do you end up throwing away produce? What you buy will have a better chance of staying out of the landfill when you begin to rely on your freezer. Here are five ways to get started:

1. Buy a bag of already washed and chopped kale, and if you only use it in cooked dishes and/or smoothies, just toss it right in the freezer when you get home. This works for spinach as well. (It doesn't work at all if you're going to eat it in a salad since when defrosted it gets mushy.)

2. Cookie sheet magic happens with most fruits and veggies that you want to use for smoothies or in cooked dishes. To freeze most things, wash and cut to the size you typically use. Blot excess water off with a paper towel, spread them out on a parchment-lined cookie sheet, and then pop the cookie sheet in the freezer. After they're frozen, put them into plastic freezer bags for later use. (You don't have to line your cookie sheet with parchment, but it does make it easier to get off the pieces. Some of the foods I've frozen this way:

   - grapes (I love eating frozen grapes.)
   - bananas (smoothies, ice cream)
   - strawberries
   - peaches
   - apples (smoothies, applesauce)
   - apricots (smoothies)
   - watermelon balls (smoothies & slushes)
   - cherries (great eaten while frozen.)
   - lemons (smoothies, slushes)
   - kale (soups, stews, stir fries, smoothies)
   - spinach (soups, stews, stir fries, smoothies)
   - green beans
   - sweet peppers (omelets, soup, stir fries, stews)
   - celery (sauté for anything you use celery in)
   - onions (sauté for anything you use onions in)
   - carrots (I just freeze baby carrots whole. I like to make glazed carrots or toss them in soups, sauces or smoothies.)

3. A treat with frozen bananas is to dip them in melted, dark chocolate (70% or higher) and

refreeze ... good for your health and fabulous for that chocolate craving! (Eat frozen)

4. Can't possibly go through a loaf of bread in time? Open the bag, fan out the slices, set in the freezer. Once frozen, put the loaf back together and seal the bag. You won't have to jackhammer the pieces apart ever again!

I'm sure there are others, so experiment! Is there something that you love, but that you end up tossing because you don't use enough of it? Try freezing it. One thing you should never freeze is a potato. They turn to absolute mush.

There you have it--tips to help your budget, your health and the landfill!

gratitude

This one is easy, give thanks for the meal or snack you are about to eat. It's an easy way to step into an attitude of gratitude which leads to greater life satisfaction. You will also become more mindful of what you are choosing to eat, and mindfulness leads to making better choices.

I had a little trouble building this habit, so I made an attractive sign on my computer, bought a little frame and put it right in the middle of my dining room table. It reminds me to take a moment to be grateful *and* mindful.

To get a printable, color copy of mine, email me at info@healthworkskc.com.

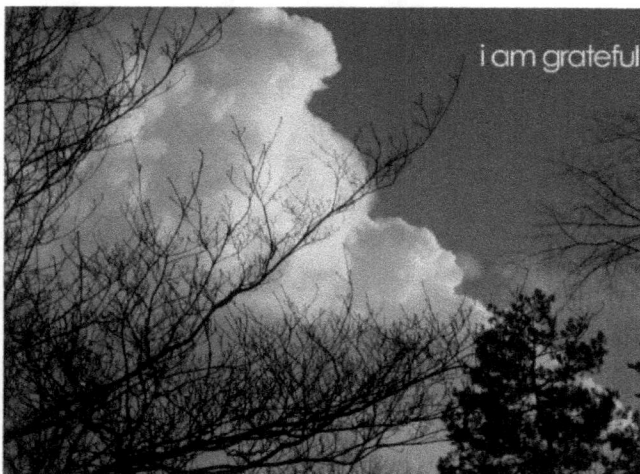

i am grateful for today

who controls
your taste buds?

Processed foods are deadly, but for some reason, they just won't stay off my radar this year. No matter where I turn I see articles about them. I was contracted to teach two classes about cravings and was asked to facilitate a 10-Day Detox group. Today I received an email with the heading, 'The 7 Deadly Truths of Sugar' and another a few weeks ago that said, "Sugar is the New Nicotine!" Last, but certainly not least, I recently had a run-in with junk foods disrupting my healthy eating plan. (I'm back on track, staying prepared and so far, I'm not experiencing cravings at all!)

So, exactly who *does* control your taste buds? Food companies manipulate their food using sugar, salt, and fat to increase the likelihood that you will consume more. There's even a name for it: craveability. Their goal, much like the tobacco companies' years ago, is to make their products more attractive and more addictive so that you'll consume greater quantities. This makes the shareholders happy and provides hefty bonuses to management. Research shows that sugar affects our dopamine receptors and that people addicted to sugar require ever greater amounts to reach the same level of satisfaction … and so we keep eating!

For more on how we are all victims of food giants out of control, read the book, *Salt Sugar Fat: How the*

Food Giants Hooked Us, by Michael Moss, a Pulitzer Prize winning journalist. It's a real eye-opener and you'll never look at packaged food the same.

Why is taste bud manipulation such a bad thing? All it takes is a look at the soaring costs of health care (or sick care) in our country to know that things aren't working well. Most Americans are happy to take a pill, or five or eight pills to 'solve' the symptoms they're experiencing and that makes the pharmaceutical companies happy! Physicians aren't taught much about nutrition and most won't advise something they don't understand. Even if you bring in research that shows it to be true many doctors aren't interested in hearing about it.

What if I told you that you could feel fabulous without any prescription medications*? Would you believe me? It's true for many people. What if I told you that you could most likely reverse heart disease with diet and exercise, or forget you ever had asthma? Maybe the arthritis in your hands prevents you from doing something you love--you can lessen, and often get rid of the pain when you change your diet.

So, what is deadly about processed foods? What are some of the conditions that its consumption leads to and/or exacerbates?

- High Cholesterol
- High Triglycerides
- Obesity
- Heart Disease
- Arthritis

- Diabetes (Type 2)
- Inflammation
- Aging Skin
- Asthma
- Immune System Suppression leaving your body less capable of warding off infection.
- Fatty Liver Disease
- Gout
- Hypoglycemia (low blood sugar)
- Hypertension
- Insulin Resistance
- Slowed Metabolism

By taking junk foods out of our diets long enough to reset our system, then adding back in healthy options, we can take back control of how we feel and how we age. I'm sure you've heard it before, but as we hit our 50's and 60's it really comes home to us: "It's not the length of a life, it's the quality of that life." In other words, I'm not enthralled by the idea of living to 100 unless I feel good and am able to enjoy myself.

*Don't ever stop a prescription medication, or start a new plan, without checking with your physician.

stretch

We like what we like, right? Maybe it's time to step out of your comfort zone and stretch a little. Is almond milk exactly like cow's milk? Nope. Is sushi really raw? Yep. Well, not all of it; you can buy fully cooked sushi, but you'd be missing out on some deliciousness you'd never expect to find in raw fish.

Do cooked apples with So Delicious Vanilla Creamer taste as rich and decadent as apple pie? Nope. But, the tradeoff is worth it! Five hundred to a thousand calories versus about 140 calories makes it not only worth it, but possible to eat every day if you want. (Dice an apple, microwave until tender, sprinkle with cinnamon and/or pumpkin pie spice to taste, add two tablespoons of So Delicious Vanilla Creamer. Presto! Hot apple pie!)

Try making a meatless chili or spaghetti sauce. Add in smoked paprika and Bragg® Liquid Aminos to mimic the flavor of meat. Smashed garbanzo beans can give you the texture of ground meat. If that's just too far, try boneless, skinless chicken thighs instead of red meat. You'll be surprised at how good it tastes. (Plus, if you don't tell anyone, they'll never know since it's covered in red sauce!)

Breakfast for Dinner? Research overwhelmingly shows that a plant-based diet is the best choice in reducing and preventing chronic disease. In some cases, it can totally reverse existing disease. Being the *Practical Health Coach*, I understand that few of my clients, or their families, are willing to make the choice to eliminate meat from their diets, so my approach is to encourage and support them in *reducing* their reliance on meat-centered meals.

One popular suggestion is to have breakfast for dinner. Not only can breakfast be prepared quite easily and quickly, the ingredients are often inexpensive, and done properly can be quite healthy. Hearty cooked breakfasts bring back memories of relaxing weekend mornings or spending the night at Grandma's—a nice way to ease some of the stress from a busy day!

My favorite is what I call a Scrambled Egg Omelet, with fried potatoes and fresh fruit. To make the omelet I sauté onions, add in broccoli, snow peas, mushrooms and spinach (broccoli first as it takes a bit longer to cook). While they're cooking, I whip up the eggs. After the veggies are cooked to the point that I like, I add the whipped eggs and stir until cooked. Season to taste and serve.

I cook thin sliced gold or red potatoes in a very small amount of coconut oil, over medium heat until browned on one side, then turn to brown on the other side.

Sometimes I cut and mix several fruits but if I'm in a hurry I slice and serve just one. If I've planned this out, I might have stopped at the salad bar for the veggies and fruit, then prep is simple! (See Use the Salad Bar)

If someone has to have bacon, or breakfast just

doesn't taste right without the smell of bacon cooking, crumble a half slice on top of their serving of either the omelet or the potatoes. (Buy uncured bacon either from or Whole Foods or similar source near you. Due to demand, several regular groceries are beginning to carry it as well.)

This is an inexpensive way to reduce your meal costs allowing you to use that money to buy better, grass-fed, organic meat.

gluten

It was bound to come up in the conversation, right? I put this on the list and skipped right past it while I wrote almost everything else. Do you know why? Because no one likes the idea of giving up bread, cake, pasta, pizza, donuts, sandwiches and just about every prepared food available—it seems too difficult. Along with dairy, giving up gluten is the recommendation I get the most push-back on. Clients bring in articles and quote television doctors. This is not a fun topic for me.

For fear of sending the non-research oriented into the hills, I haven't included a lot of the science here. If you're into research, I recommend reading *Non-Celiac Gluten Sensitivity Where Are We Now in 2015?* in *Practical Gastroenterology,* June 2015. It gives an in-depth overview of the current state of research into the spectrum of gluten sensitivity disorders.

I want to make sure that you know that Celiac Disease is a different condition than gluten sensitivity or intolerance. When someone has Celiac Disease their body's immune system goes on the attack and destroys the villi that line their small intestines. This destruction reduces the surface area available to absorb most nutrients and allows them to pass through the intestines and be eliminated, resulting in malnutrition, a weakened immune system and serious illness. In this section I am going to focus on gluten sensitivity/intolerance.

Where is gluten found? In wheat, rye, barley, graham, and in oats not specifically identified as gluten-free. (Oats are typically milled on the same equipment as wheat, thus contaminated.)

I encourage clients to give a gluten-free diet a try for a few months because the symptoms of gluten sensitivity/intolerance are often subtle and are things we've accepted for many years as normal. Then they add it back in. If they felt better without it, or felt worse after adding it back, they took it out of their diet completely. There are hundreds of thousands of people in the United States of America who are living proof that, not only can it be done, it can be done happily and with grace.

"This gluten free thing is just trendy. We've been eating bread and cereal since the beginning of time, why would it trouble me now?" I hear this a lot as well. One answer is that today's wheat has been bred to contain far more gluten. Why? Because gluten is what makes bread fluffy and soft. It's a stretchy protein that creates the texture we love. And, it's a cheap ingredient so it's being added to everything from soup to candy, bouillon to imitation crab. Walk through the grocery store and pick up a box or can every few feet. Unless you're in the veggie aisle, you're likely to see, under the Allergen Information: wheat. It's everywhere!

Check out your favorite restaurant's online gluten free menu. I'm certain you'll be shocked to find that even most French fries have gluten. Our bodies are being inundated with an ingredient that humans have never been able to digest, but used to only get in small quantities. Our immune systems are overwhelmed and are responding to the invaders exactly as they were designed to.

Here are some of the symptoms of gluten sensitivity or intolerance that we often mistake for aging or hormonal changes:

- digestive problems including: gas, bloating, diarrhea and even constipation
- Keratosis Pilaris, that chicken skin look on the back of your arms
- chronic fatigue or fibromyalgia, general fatigue or brain fog, sometimes after eating a meal containing gluten
- autoimmune disease
- hormonal imbalance
- headaches
- joint inflammation or pain
- problems with balance
- anxiety, depression, mood swings and ADD.

Dr. Amy Myers wrote, "An article published in 2001 states that for those with celiac disease or gluten sensitivity eating gluten just once a month increased the relative risk of death by 600%.[x]"

For those who are willing to give it a try, there are multitudes of guides online, but I'll add my recommendation: Don't replace regular cookies or cakes with gluten free versions except on special occasions. There are a lot of gluten free alternatives, but they are often loaded with ultra-refined flours and extra sugar. Buyer/baker beware! Read labels and look for whole grains while avoiding sugar and refined starches.

kick soda to the curb

You want to kick the soda habit but so far you haven't had any luck. There are many reasons to do so from the acid in diet soda having the same effect on your teeth as methamphetamines, to it increasing your risk of pancreatic cancer. Research has linked soda to obesity, stroke, diabetes and osteoporosis.

Let's see if a step-by-step approach will do the trick. First you need to determine if you like drinking soda for the fizz, the sweetness or both. If it's for the fizz, you can solve it by drinking one of the many varieties of sparkling water. I'm talking about the sparkling water that is water and maybe flavor if necessary. There's lemon, lime, grapefruit, cranberry, orange, etc. They have no added chemicals, no sugar or artificial sweeteners.

If you drink soda for the sweetness you might want to try eating fruit. An ice cold serving of fresh pineapple, clementine, watermelon or crunchy apple would address the sweet craving and be so good for you!

If you're like me, it's both sweet and fizz. I solved my habit by making a delicious combo of 2 ounces of 100% cherry, orange or pomegranate juice, 2 ounces of kombucha* and 12 ounces of sparkling water. It's sweet, tart and fizzy and I absolutely love it! This combo is really good for you too. You're adding in water, fruit juice and tons of nutrition, and probiotics from the kombucha. A trifecta of goodness!

Some people aren't big fans of kombucha so they enjoy the juice and sparkling water without it. Do what works for you!

Another favorite recipe for cold refreshment during the hot summer months, and to give you the fizz you miss is Sparkling Lemonade: In a large glass, combine the juice of one small lemon, stevia to taste (I like NuNaturals Liquid Stevia) and one 12-ounce can of lemon LaCroix sparkling water. Add ice and enjoy! (Limeade is also delicious! Substitute lime sparkling water and lime juice.)

You can have pint jars with lemon juice and stevia already mixed in your fridge. then all you have to do is take one out, pour in a can of sparkling water, add ice and gently stir.

Reward yourself for making a healthy choice by creating a drink that's as nice to look at as it is to enjoy by adding a dash of pomegranate or cherry juice, and for that extra special feeling add a couple of frozen strawberries to the jar. Lovely!

We're on a journey and sometimes the choices we make are difficult. For a lot of my clients and students giving up their Diet Coke was one of the hardest. These recipes made it easier for many of them; I hope it works for you.
Side note: Did you know that Coca Cola saw their first decline in sales in decades? Not to worry. They've entered into the lucrative sparkling water category that's primarily been led by La Croix and Canada Dry.

* Kombucha is fermented green tea. It has 40 calories per 8 ounces. The brand I like best is G.T.'s Kombucha™ and can be found at grocery stores nationwide. Its health benefits are made possible because of its probiotics and variety of enzymes and organic acids. Loaded with B vitamins, kombucha has been around for over 2000 years. and has been credited with curing/preventing cancer, arthritis, building the immune system, detoxifying the body and aiding in digestion. Bet you can't say that about your soda pop!

watermelon: it's not just for summer!

When it's not the official watermelon season some of my sustainably-minded friends might give me grief, but those little 'personal' watermelons are very tasty at almost any time of year. (I prefer to call them snack size since I consider any watermelon my 'personal' watermelon—size matters not!)

Sweet, crisp and cold watermelon is my idea of perfection. Don't take my word for it; here are some facts about this amazing green striped orb:

Watermelon has more lycopene than tomatoes—20mg per six cup serving. Why do you care? Lycopene is an incredible antioxidant! Researchers have found evidence that shows by including it in your diet you can positively impact heart disease, cancer (most notably lung, stomach, breast, cervix and prostate), diabetes and osteoporosis. Toss in a side of anti-aging support and watermelon is a big winner!

Because watermelon's antioxidants corral a bunch of free radicals it reduces the damage they can cause. Damage that includes the inflammation of arthritis, severity of asthma attacks and the stickiness of cholesterol which leads to atherosclerosis.

One serving supports lower blood pressure and insulin

sensitivity, and is loaded with Vitamin A, C, B6, B1, potassium and magnesium offering strong support for your immune system.

Fun facts: Watermelon is a vegetable that belongs to the same family as pumpkin, cucumber and squash … who knew? Due to its high water content (92% water) explorers used watermelons as canteens.

Watermelon is gaining a reputation for its versatility; add it to salads or smoothies, create frozen summer treats or, if you're like me, just eat it cold and crisp from the fridge!

After years of experience, even I can't pick out the perfect watermelon every time and it's disappointing to be looking forward to that crisp goodness only to find that the texture is weird or that it lacks flavor. In that case, I cut it into chunks, put it on my trusty cookie sheet and freeze it for use in smoothies or slushes.

use the salad bar
Get Yourself a Prep Cook

The number one thing that stops people from preparing a healthy meal at home is the prep work. All that washing, peeling and dicing is not what people want to do when they get home from work.

One solution would be to hire a prep cook, but most people can't afford a kitchen guru. I've figured out the next best thing: use the services of someone else's prep cook. The salad bar at your favorite grocery store is the perfect place to find most of the ingredients you'll need to create a delicious meal, and they're already prepared!

There are no signs up at the salad bar that say, 'SALADS ONLY!' Go ahead and load up on washed, peeled, sliced and diced onions, celery, carrots, beets, cabbage, mushrooms, snow peas, bean sprouts, spinach, kale—whatever you need. Going for a sweet dish instead of savory? They have cranberries, melon, strawberries, pineapples, grapes, nuts and more!

The per-pound price might be higher, but you'll save a bundle by not buying the full-sized package or bundle of ingredients that you don't need and often never use. After all, how many mung bean sprouts can you use in a few days? This choice also keeps a lot of food out of the landfill.

Here's an extra tip: While you're there, pick up a salad for tomorrow's lunch!

rice at the ready

One of the best things you can do to streamline your dinner prep, and reduce the likelihood you'll go through the nearest drive-thru, is to always have a batch of cooked rice on hand. This simple step will provide you with opportunities galore!

Pilaf … Your way!
This is something you can make all your own. You don't need a recipe! Using the salad bar as your prep cook, toss in whatever veggies and/or fruit appeals to you. My favorite is a Mediterranean-flavored pilaf with spinach, garlic, onion, tomato and chickpeas tossed with olive oil, balsamic (lightly), oregano and basil. If you eat dairy, a touch of feta cheese would be lovely.

And, for a delicious sweet pilaf drizzle walnut oil and cinnamon pear balsamic vinegar over rice, diced apples, carrots, celery and walnuts. If the cinnamon flavor isn't strong enough, sprinkle on a bit more.

For pilafs, just add what you think will work. Experiment with oils (I like olive or walnut oil) and then add spices to flavor it. For a Southwest feel, add chili powder, peppers, onions and cumin. If you're craving Italian, add garlic, onion, parsley, basil, tomatoes, lemon, a touch of fresh parmesan and olive oil.

When creating sweet pilafs, I often blend fresh pineapple with yellow mustard and honey (in my NutriBullet®) to create a healthy twist on honey mustard. It is DELICIOUS!! Just play with amounts. Start with the pineapple; give it a squirt of mustard and a teaspoon of honey. Blend, taste, adjust, blend, taste, adjust. Be adventurous!

You can dress pilaf with whatever you like including, Asian style, Italian, Balsamic, Russian or French dressing. You can create your own dressing by combining oil and vinegar, soy sauce and spices. Bottled dressings often have a ton of additives or sugar so I usually make my own.

You can add just about anything to rice to make it a delicious side dish: onions, carrots, peas, peppers, radishes, edamame, beans, chickpeas, beets, mushrooms, bean sprouts, tomatoes, dried cranberries, nuts, sunflower seeds, sesame seeds, peanuts ...

breakfast is
for champions!

It's critical that you end your overnight fast, and fuel your body for the coming day, with good, solid nutrition. I've heard so many people say they feel hungrier if they eat. I'm going to guess that they begin their day with sugary cereal, donuts or muffins. This is your opportunity to end that!

The key to a great start is protein, so start with an egg, nut butter, lean meat, beans or low-fat dairy. Plant-based protein is my easy solution. I drink a Juice Plus+® Complete Shake in the morning because it tastes terrific and has the perfect balance of protein, carbs, fiber and fat. Even a healthy fruit smoothie can leave you hungry if you don't have protein and fat in it to slow down the release of sugar into your system.

One way to add a healthy breakfast to your daily routine is to decide what you're going to have and make it consistent. If you love eggs, have them two or three days a week. On the other days have a smoothie, yogurt or nut butter with an all-fruit spread on whole grain toast. Or pick something plant-based and have it almost every day.

Fast, Easy, Healthy
Make the same smoothie for the week. Buy the ingredients, measure and freeze into individual bags,

and all you have to do in the morning is toss it in the blender with your choice of liquid and you're good to go.

If you choose the nut butter option, make sure to measure so that you don't kill it on the calories. I love PBJ on a Lundberg Brown Rice Cake!

Be careful when you buy yogurt. It can be loaded with sugar or artificial sweeteners. To avoid that, buy a large container of plain yogurt and a bag of frozen unsweetened berries. Thaw the berries and combine with the yogurt. Transfer to single serve containers.

Do you love bananas? Add a mashed banana to plain yogurt, sprinkle with a tablespoon of chopped walnuts and you have a powerhouse breakfast!

Hard boiled eggs are one way to add protein to your morning and are something that most people are comfortable having for breakfast. Cook up several at a time so that they're handy.

These breakfasts are all under five minutes in the morning and can even be taken with you on your commute. With a little planning, you can make your body happy by giving it topnotch fuel.

Starting your day with nutritious food is a good first step on your journey to better health.

play with your food
Here's Permission!

It can be a lot of fun to experiment with foods you've never tried. By doing a bit of research online you'll find recipes and suggestions on how best to prepare just about anything. Take time to read some of the comments and you are likely to find helpful tips that will turn the original recipe into one that's perfect for your family.

By adding in new foods, you're adding in the unique nutrient delivery systems we discussed in the beginning, and increasing the likelihood of getting the nourishment you need. So, not only will you be adding new flavors to your menu, you'll be adding a whole different package of nutrients. Variety is important!

I was asked what I thought about black rice during a class, but hadn't heard of it. I found it at a Trader Joe's and purchased a bag. (If you can't find it near you, it's available on Amazon.) After giving it a rinse, I cooked it following the directions on the package. It took a bit longer to cook than indicated, but when it was done and I tasted it, I was transported! It has an almost creamy risotto-like texture, and is a beautiful purple color. It has the perfect bit of crunch. Just a sprinkle of salt and it was delicious.

The nutritional information comes as no surprise; black rice is loaded with nutrients. Whenever a whole food is dark in color, it's usually the healthier choice over its paler family members. Black rice is no exception. It contains a large number of anthocyanins, reducing the risk of heart attacks by preventing the buildup of plaque. Anthocyanins are also better at controlling cholesterol levels than any other food supplement[xi].

Black rice is a nutritional powerhouse! I highly recommend adding it to your diet. If you have kids, they're bound to love it. It turns a dark purple when cooked. What kid doesn't like dark purple food? It's probably too creamy to use for pilaf, but would be great as a warm or cold whole grain cereal. Is oatmeal boring? This might be a huge hit in the morning! (By the way, that's why kids love green smoothies … they're green!)

pizza and beer

Indulge! What can this possibly have to do with a healthy lifestyle you ask? Well, if pizza and beer is food that you love, and if you're not an alcoholic, then go for it! Yep! Go for it!

I admit, there's a catch. You can only go for it 10-20% of the time. The rest of the time you have to eat real, healthy foods. You don't have to achieve the 80% today, or even tomorrow, but it should be your goal.

It's much easier to eat healthy meals most of the time if you know that on Friday night or Sunday afternoon you can eat pizza and drink beer--right?

This practice works well for most of my clients. It helps to know that you're not giving up the food you love forever. Relax, go out with friends and have a good time without worrying about the food! Just make it your 20%. Of course, if you're gluten or dairy free you still have some restrictions, indulge where you can.

A great way to work up to the 80/20 rule is to pick the meals for which you can easily maintain healthy choices, then relax with the others. If breakfast and lunch are easy, but dinner is a challenge, focus on breakfast and lunch until healthy versions of them are second nature. Once this occurs, move on to creating healthy dinners, one weeknight at a time.

In no time you'll be easily following the 80/20 rule and on your way to 90/10!

go ahead
and try a detox

It feels great to have energy, sleep better and lose weight! When you're in the middle of a detox, it's hard to even think back to how you felt before you started. If you think you'll go crazy without your favorite foods, think again. For almost every person who sticks with it for the first two days, it's turned out to be easy. Some thought they'd go crazy without coffee ... Again, pretty easy. (Although, it gets added back in fairly quickly once the detox is over.) And every single person who joined one of my groups thought that sugar would be IMPOSSIBLE! (I think that every time, but in reality, and with good preparation, it is hardly a blip on the radar.)

The good things that happen?
- Great sleep
- High energy levels
- Working out is easier
- Better circulation
- Glowing skin
- Weight/Inches lost. (If you also watch your portion size, you'll lose more, but the most important thing is to eat the right foods.)
- Improved focus

Here are some testimonials from a few of my group members:

" ... the best gift I've ever given myself. Thanks so much Nancy, I'm telling all my friends!"

"I have enjoyed the 10-day detox and cannot

believe the 10 days have passed. I feel amazing! I was a little worried beginning the program that I would have major cravings, but I found it easy."

"I am going to continue on with the program, being mindful of what I eat. Everyone should do this detox. Nancy, thank you for a great 10 days!"

They each lost a minimum of 5-6 pounds. Some lost 10 pounds in 10 days!

I follow Dr. Mark Hyman's *10-Day Detox Diet* because it can truly change your medical status by reducing your:

- Blood Sugar
- Blood Pressure
- Cholesterol
- Weight
- Inflammation

I believe in supporting people in improving the quality of their lives. This isn't sissy stuff ... it's really important stuff ... stuff that can totally change how you feel as you age. The conditions this reverses are conditions that can stop you in your tracks and leave you barely able to get around, even kill you. You can begin to live again.

If you want to do it on your own, get the book. If you want extra support visit my website: nancyoglesby.com or email me at info@healthworkskc.com.

I would love to support you on your journey! It's rewarding when you find out how easy it is to regulate your blood sugar and get off the sugar merry-go-round for good! You can do anything for ten days, right?

be good to your heart

Chia! These little, bitty seeds pack a wallop! 1oz. (1T + 1/2t) has 9g fat, 4g protein (high quality containing all essential amino acids except for taurine), 12g carbohydrate, 11g fiber; 1620mg Omega-6, 4915mg Omega-3, 18% DV of calcium and it's also high in phosphorous, and manganese. Chia also contains zinc, potassium, copper, niacin, folic acid and magnesium[xii].

All that nutrition is packed into a tiny seed that's tasteless! That means you can add it to almost anything without affecting the taste. Go ahead, sprinkle it on salads, cereal and yogurt or blend it up in your smoothie.

So, what are the health claims? The Aztecs ate chia seeds for energy. It is reported to be mildly anti-inflammatory, slows the digestion of carbohydrates helping to regulate blood sugar, lowers bad and raises good cholesterol, aids in weight loss and helps to control cravings. Because it's loaded with antioxidants it aids in the prevention of heart disease and hypertension and should be included in any anti-aging strategy. It also aids in hydration and is great for your skin

As if all that isn't enough, unlike flax seed, chia doesn't need to be ground to get the benefits, making it easier and faster to use; and it doesn't need careful handling because it doesn't get rancid due to its high levels of antioxidants. I've read that you can keep them for two years.

Chia seeds turn liquid into a gel-like substance that surrounds the seed. It makes a fantastic base for a raw pudding. I got the following recipe from Raw Foods Witch[xiii]:

1/4c chia seeds, 1.5c almond or other nut milk, dash of vanilla, sweetener of choice (I love pure maple syrup). Put all ingredients in a glass jar, shake to mix and refrigerate overnight ... Voila! Pudding!

curb cravings

When cravings hit, they usually hit HARD! Why?

Physical cravings

Sometimes it's because we've been working hard and the glucose from our food has been depleted from carrying energy to our brains and muscles. When the glucose gets low, this type of craving occurs. We often feel sluggish, lose our concentration, experience headaches, get the shakes or have some serious hunger pangs.

Dehydration, or simple thirst, can show up as a sugar craving, so if you are craving sugar, try drinking a glass of water and waiting 15 minutes. Another way that physical cravings occur is to balance out your system. If you regularly crave sugar, reduce your salt intake. If you regularly crave chips, reduce sugar.

You might not feel like you're eating a lot of salt. But, most processed and restaurant foods are loaded with it. Even if you don't pour it on with a shaker you are probably getting a lot. And, if you just thought, "But I don't eat a lot of sugar, I much prefer chips," your body is getting a lot more sugar than you think. Sugar isn't just in candy bars and cookies. Chips, corn, potatoes, rice, pasta, bread ... they all turn to sugar in your body.

There's one more thing that's all sugar. Most people think that bars keep salty snacks on hand because they make you thirsty and you'll drink more alcohol.

While that's true, the reason salty snacks work so well is that they increase your craving for sugar, and alcohol is just that. Your body will do what it can to stay in balance.

Emotional cravings

This type of craving occurs when we use food to mask our feelings. It's easy to do and we don't always recognize it. For example, it's Saturday afternoon, you're home alone with only household chores on your horizon. Yuck! Instead, you go to the kitchen and get a donut, cookie or ice cream and then a few minutes later you're back in the kitchen looking for some chips. You're bored and uninterested in what's on the horizon so you choose something more pleasurable.

What to do? Stopping the donut/chip cycle is easier said than done. Any type of craving behavior requires awareness. You need to recognize when it typically occurs and how you're feeling at the time. Keeping a small notebook or using an app like *My Fitness Pal* to track your food and emotions is incredibly helpful in this process. Looking back over the information will give you strategies for when/how to implement the ideas at the end of this chapter.

Boredom isn't the only thing that sends us to the cookie jar; there are the culprits you might expect, like anger, sadness, envy, fear, embarrassment, disgust, shame or frustration, but there are also emotions that might surprise you on the list: happiness, celebration, enthusiasm, love and joy. These are a few examples of the many emotions we humans experience.

For some, finding the exact emotion could be the key to recognizing when you are in danger of falling into the spiral of emotional eating. Google 'list of emotions' and find the ones that fit your situation.

Be prepared for cravings by having healthy choices available and by limiting the availability of unhealthy ones.

Examples of healthy choices include:

- An ounce (1/4 cup) of nuts and a piece of fruit or mini box of raisins.

- Healthy trail mix with a lot of nuts and small amount of dried fruit. I make my own from the bulk bins to get the blend I want. It's easy to have with you, or leave in your car, regardless of the outside temperature.

- Celery and peanut butter (Buy peanut butter without added sugar.)

- Hummus & cucumber slices (or any fresh veggies you enjoy)

- Craving sugar? Eat sweet veggies like carrots and sweet peppers.

- 1 piece of Dark Chocolate (70% or higher, 70-100 calories). Paired with fruit this seems like a decadent indulgence, but it's actually a healthy choice!

- Larabar (nuts, fruit, dates ... that's it!) They are calorie rich, but when you're out of trail mix and need something on the run, this is a good choice.

- PBJ--yep! A peanut butter and jelly sandwich, grown-up style! Use whole grain bread, no-sugar-added organic peanut butter (or almond butter) and either fresh fruit or all-fruit jam.

When you've identified your craving as emotional, try going for a walk or to the gym for a good workout. Exercise has been proven to lower stress, so when you're done you just might have beaten that craving! If you're still hungry, at least you will have added to your energy-expenditure, and you've had time to think about what kind of healthy snack you'll have instead of the junk food you almost picked up.

Most people have cravings; they're not always a bad thing. Sometimes a craving is your body's way of getting what it needs whether it's nutrition, comfort, release or the need to relax. Potato chips only give temporary comfort and almost no nutrition—Understanding what we really need is the key to resolving our seemingly out-of-control cravings.

add in greens

What leafy greens did you eat today? Greens, as a category, are incredibly easy to find, are available in great variety and are packed with nutrition. You can find locally grown greens almost everywhere year-round, and you can easily add them to smoothies, omelets, stir fries, salads and soups. (See Get Sneaky for more ideas.) Don't judge all greens on the basis of one. If you don't like one variety of kale, you might like another or the baby version.

Greens are one of the best healthy additions you can make to your lifestyle. They contain vitamins and thousands of phytonutrients. They improve circulation, purify the blood, strengthen the immune system, reduce cardiovascular disease and diabetes risk, protect against macular degeneration ... and they lift the spirit.

I am really lucky because my neighbor has a HUGE collard green patch and one day she gave me a bag of just-picked goodness. I added some curly kale that I had on hand, and cooked it up in a quarter cup of water. When it was tender I chopped it up, added some chopped onion and broccoli and sautéed it all together. When the onion was tender I poured a scrambled egg over the top and cooked it to perfection ... Served with a slice of ice cold watermelon it was heaven on a plate! By the way, the egg was from a different neighbor's sister's homestead. Am I spoiled or what?

For lunch I added the remaining greens (and cooking water) to my leftover homemade split pea soup. There was no way I was throwing out all of that nutrition! I chose fresh peaches and a handful of cherries for a side.

One of the easiest ways I've found to get people to add in variety is to put a handful of mixed baby greens into a salad mix that they already enjoy. It eases you into experiencing a new texture and flavor.

Whatever ways you find to make greens a regular part of your diet, this is one addition your body will thank you for making!

tell me i can't

Tell me I can't and I'll work harder to prove that I can. It's just who I am. I've found a way to put that rebellious streak to good use: When a food calls to me, candy or potato chips, and I give in and eat too much, I buy another one and put it on the table where I'll see it all day, every day. Every time I walk through my house I see it, give it the evil eye and say, "YOU will not win this battle!"

It works. I've found that I do better when I know the enemy and look it right in the eye. Having it where I can see it there's little chance of a sneak attack. Some examples from over the years:

I hung a donut on a pushpin in my studio in the 80's. It was labeled the 'First Donut I Didn't Eat.' When I left two years later the donut was still on the pushpin looking exactly as it had the day I put it up there. Yuck!

Years ago I quit smoking cold turkey. I had a two-pack-a-day habit, and I quit with a carton of cigarettes in the glove compartment of my car. 100% success! Why? Someone told me I'd never make it.

I bought Easter candy on sale, ate several pieces while in a total fog, came out of it and put the rest of the candy in a dish on my dining room table. There was no way that candy was going to bring me down. Where is it today? Dusty!

I stared the enemy right in the eye and claimed my power! Exhilarating!

(As an aside, I can't tell you I'd be able to walk by my mom's fried chicken but since I'm the only one who makes it anymore I'm pretty safe … from buying pastured chicken to preparing it is a long time to get over a craving. Occasionally I go through the process and it tastes a little bit like heaven!)

It's important to learn the difference between foods you love and foods that trigger actual binges. You win against food addictions one battle at a time. As you learn and eliminate the foods that trigger binges and cravings the enemy army becomes smaller and weaker while you become stronger both physically and psychologically.

Once you know the enemy you can make conscious choices to eat the foods you love. I find that just knowing a specific food has the capacity to cause massive cravings keeps me clear of it 99% of the time. I also know that when I do choose to eat it I need to be on top of my game to prevent a landslide of unhealthy eating.

The moral of the story: Know your enemy; Find your fighter's stance; **Claim your power!**

shop local

I am grateful for the people at the grassroots level that are choosing to grow their food and mine; urban farmers, family farmers, beekeepers, herbalists ... those who are doing things the old fashioned way trying to heal the land and our families. These folks are leading the charge to freedom from poisons deemed 'safe,' including chemical fertilizers, pesticides, genetic modifications, growth hormones, antibiotics and feed that is laced with all of the above.

The food from people that care is energetically superior to that which is factory farmed. There is true love and commitment involved in farming organically and sustainably. That is the energy that's in the food from a farmers market ... love, and sweat, and tradition. Have a little of that with your dinner!

There are many places to purchase grass fed, grass finished beef and pastured chickens. They are usually more expensive, but as demand grows, prices keep getting a little bit lower. This brings me to one of my favorite Michael Pollan quotes: "Eat food. Not too much. Mostly plants." Eat the best that you can afford. Learn to replace some meat entrees with bean dishes for health and to keep costs down. (Chili with beans, bean soup, salads with beans and black bean burgers are just a few choices.)

Many urban areas are lucky to have farmers bring what's been ordered to a central location for pickup, or they attend farmers markets and bring pre-ordered items along. Check out Local Harvest for growers in your area. In the KC area you can download a directory of members at KC Food Circle.

Most of the farmers I've met are full of advice for how to use their products; many offering plants and recipes. There are a growing number of new businesses springing up to teach homeowners how to cultivate their yards for organic food production. Edible landscaping is a fantastic way to save money and teach children where food really comes from!

No room to garden or the critters get into everything? Do you have a brown thumb? Try a Tower Garden® from Juice Plus+. I was never able to grow veggies in a regular garden. When I tried, and the plants started to grow, the squirrels and rabbits decimated every single plant before anything was ripe.

Then I ordered a Tower Garden®, paid for it in twelve installments and for the first time, had fresh tomatoes, cucumbers, watermelon, okra, celery, bell peppers and rosemary. I love it! I caught a squirrel on it one day, sprinkled the base with cayenne pepper and as long as I keep pepper on the base, they stay away. The rabbits aren't able to get up on it.

As I sit here editing one last time, I have to add that it's winter and my Tower is now inside adding a sunny glow to my office. Once an hour, for fifteen minutes, it sounds like a lovely rain shower as the water flows over the roots of the kale, lettuce, Swiss chard, sweet peas, basil and arugula that is flourishing indoors! I have had freshly picked kale to add to my smoothies in the morning and to have in a delicious Kale Salad at dinner. Freshly-grown produce in the Midwestern winter ... Heaven!

Tower Gardens® are aeroponic, with no dirt, no weeds and no bending. Now I enjoy fresh veggies all year. They work great on patios and balconies, and even in the garden.

There's a little bit of a learning curve when you first get your Tower Garden®, but this brown thumb gardener had tons of produce in the first year. They're durable and built to last for years!

I can step outside, pick a tomato and eat it right then and there because there are absolutely no chemicals on it! For more information, visit my Tower Garden website: www.nancyoglesby.towergarden.com

Still not growing your own? No problem! Thank a food activist and visit a farmers market in your town.

relapse prevention

I've had a long history with friends and loved ones in AA, and I was close to certification as an Addictions Counselor several years ago, so I know a thing or two about addiction and relapse. When it comes to sugar and refined flour (sugar in a different form) I recognize an addiction when I see one. I am addicted to sugar.

One night, this normally healthy eater found herself in a sugar stupor after having eaten fifteen ... one at a time ... mini Milky Ways®. Fifteen! I admit it had been a difficult few days, but typically, if I found myself in an emotional eating frame of mind, I would head for the carrots, celery, romaine or apples. This was a full-on relapse into the old unhealthy sugar jar!

I don't keep candy in my house. This was in the house because of an outreach program in which participants put together Easter baskets for people who wouldn't otherwise receive them and I was putting together a couple of baskets. Of course I thought I'd just have a couple of those little minis-- yeah, right! How quickly we forget that we are just one mini Milky Way® away from a date with a sugar coma!

I did what any self-respecting addict in recovery would do: I accepted responsibility and acknowledged my mistake, and then I created a Relapse Prevention Plan. I highly recommend it. Work toward identifying your triggers so that BEFORE you jump into a full-on frenzy with candy, potato chips or ice cream you recognize what's happening and go directly to your plan to prevent it. It's an especially helpful tool when you've gone a long time without having a problem and suddenly find yourself heading into the danger zone.

Here is my Relapse Prevention Plan. Use it for ideas on how to create your own:

- Check my Nourishment Menu. This is a menu of things I enjoy doing that nourish me in other ways. For me it includes: bubble bath, walk the dogs, create a graphic using a motivational quote, look through my photos for pictures that would work well in my blog, dance, exercise or do yoga, go into my studio and draw or paint.
- Remember that it is an addiction and that I'm not capable of having just one regardless of how hard I try to convince myself that I can.
- Call my relapse buddy. Set this up ahead of time! File them under Relapse so you don't have to try to remember who to call.
- Have faith that the craving will go away.
- Journal about the situation.
- Do something physical: Dance, walk, exercise … whatever.
- Brush your teeth.
- Give yourself a pedicure.
- Limit salty foods since they lead to the body wanting to balance itself with sugar. Don't claim a spot on that seesaw!
- Eat carrots … even if I don't want to … do it anyway.

So, you fell off the wagon. Trust me, it happens a lot! What can you do to get back on track? Focus on your recovery pledge.

My recovery pledge

I will:

- Become aware of the behavior that signals potential problems.
- Ask a friend or two to be my relapse buddies.
- Go through my relapse prevention plan before I head to my substance of choice.

If you'd like, share your ideas for relapse prevention. They might end up in my next book, along with your name! Please send them to me via the contact page on my website www.nancyoglesby.com or email me at info@healthworkskc.com

moderation

How can you impact your health and the health of the planet, along with everyone and everything on it? Practice moderation.

Wow! Simple.

To see a significant improvement in your health and impact the world at the same time, moderate your intake of processed foods and increase the amount of whole foods you eat. First decide what processed foods you want to keep in your diet. It can change from week to week. Go with your desires.

Do you salivate at the idea of freshly baked bread? Eat it. Savor it. Rejoice in its perfection ... Once a week. Is your idea of heaven apple pie? McDonald's® Quarter Pounder® with Cheese? French fries? A juicy steak cooked to perfection? French toast slathered with butter and syrup? Barbeque? A crazy bleu cheese-bacon-double cheeseburger? Eat it. Savor it. Rejoice in its perfection ... But choose carefully and only indulge occasionally. Moderation.

Americans have forgotten the life-giving nature of whole foods: blueberries and strawberries, oranges and melon, lettuce mixes, red peppers, radishes, celery and carrots, beautifully colorful vegetables; the colors of the rainbow nurture our bodies and give us incredible energy.

Great news! It doesn't require much effort to create a healthy meal. Most grocery stores have salad bars loaded with whole foods. Just pass up the heavy, creamy, pasta salads in favor of fresh vegetables and fruit. Top your colorful salad with some beans and dress with vinegar, olive oil, some seasonings and a scoop of sunflower seeds or almonds. DINNER!

The United States has become a nation of people eating with abandon whether hungry or not, choosing to ignore the high price of their choices: poor health physically, psychologically and monetarily, and a planet that cannot sustain the destruction.

Here's to good health!

keep the junk out

This is so much easier said than done, but if you don't bring junk into the house you can't eat it at midnight or for breakfast or that lazy snack while dinner is cooking. And if you don't eat it, your kids won't eat it either.

I don't expect you to never eat junk food; just don't make it an easy habit to have. If potato chips are your favorite junk food, then buy a single-serving bag (or two) every once in a while. (Note that I didn't say every day or two.) Plan to have them at a specific time and savor them!

Many people stock up on things because it's cheaper to buy a big container (of chips, cookies, candy, ice cream) than a small one, but if you eat it all in a day and a half, it wasn't really cheaper.

Take a look in your kitchen cabinets and count the number of foods you've got that are instant fixes. Now think about what would happen if that food wasn't there. It's true that you might actually get in your car and drive to the store, but the likelihood is that the desire would pass or you would eat or drink something already there instead. If it's not there, you can't put it in your mouth!

One of the easiest, healthiest alternatives to junk food snacking is to have healthy snacks available. Roasted and spiced chickpeas, nuts, ready-to-eat veggies with a healthy dip such as guacamole, hummus or salsa, 100% whole grain crackers, brown rice cakes (Lundberg is my favorite) with a smear of 100% peanut butter and a touch of all-fruit spread, peanut butter on apples or celery, Cuties, bananas ... the list is endless (and healthy)!

It's much more difficult to break a habit unless you replace it with another one, so in order to avoid leaving a vacuum, I recommend that you have some healthy alternatives on hand. (Get ideas from Curb Your Cravings.)

As you break the junk food/processed food habits your taste buds will come alive. You'll be amazed at the sweet deliciousness of an apple smeared with peanut butter. It will make you think of a caramel apple but without the sugar, artificial colors or flavors. Fresh food becomes delicious!

portion control

As much as I hate it, counting calories works. It works especially well when you're eating whole, real food because your body is getting all of the phytonutrients found in whole foods and so it responds better than when you're choosing a lot of your calories from processed foods.

A natural byproduct of calorie counting is that you learn the portion you should be eating. Here is some interesting information on portions:

- The USDA MyPlate Guidelines[xiv] recommends a total of 5.5 ounces of protein/day for those consuming a 2000 calorie diet. That includes meat, eggs, nuts, seeds and beans. An average-sized burger, at a quarter of a pound, leaves you with only 1.5 ounces left for the entire day.
- The USDA recommends no more than 10 grams of added sugar per day, (USDA.gov) and while it appears that McDonald's® eliminated the Supersized drink, their large drink (I couldn't find the ounces listed on the website) has a whopping 81 grams of sugar according to their online nutrition calculator.[xv] Burger King and Taco Bell offer a 40-oz. option with Mountain Dew coming in at 145 grams of sugar, again from Taco Bell's online nutrition calculator[xvi]. McDonald's *extra small* serving of Coca-Cola® has 33 grams of sugar!
- It is recommended that we get 7-13 servings of fruits & vegetables each day but Americans are

barely getting 2-3, and much of our fruit intake is in the form of juice rather than whole fruit. (Jelly doesn't count!) Fruits and veggies are the most amazing things! They heal the body and create healthy DNA, and we are not eating them, and our kids aren't eating them either. If we want to feel good we need to get on track and add in fruits and veggies!

- The actual portion size of cooked spaghetti is one cup. The actual portion size of cooked steak or chicken is 3 ounces. The actual portion size of a bowl of cereal is ¾ of a cup. If you measure and weigh you will be shocked.

So, what should your plate look like? I've seen portion sizes compared to decks of cards or golf and tennis balls, but I really do like the MyPlate visual. Half of your plate should have fruits and vegetables while whole grains and lean protein make up the other half, every single meal, including breakfast! (Smoothies make this easy!)

For portion control I suggest calorie counting to see what the calorie cost of food truly is. We have been brainwashed into thinking that a restaurant dish should be huge. We boast about the size of the entrée we got at dinner the night before, all the while we are getting less and less healthy.

snack before dinner

The best way to give in to that raging hunger when you come in the door after a long day is to have a vegetable tray in the fridge ready to put out on the table or kitchen counter for your snacking pleasure. It's a terrific way to get family members to eat their veggies and it will help everyone to eat less of the heavier items in the meal.

Another option is to throw together a salad, sit down with everyone to enjoy the fresh food, catch up on the day and then go off to do what needs doing, coming back together for the meal a bit later. Make sure your dressing has healthy fat in it, otherwise your salad won't have much staying power, nor will you be able to absorb the fat-soluble vitamins (A, D, E and K).

Try a nice bowl of clear soup before you begin preparing your meal, especially in the winter. It allows time to breathe and relax before beginning. This can be as simple as bouillon or broth with a few snipped chives. I've been known to toss in some spinach leaves or frozen peas to add a bit of substance as well.

Fresh fruit is another option, but I always feel as though that's best left for dessert.

Whatever you choose to do, share the experience with family or friends. There's absolutely no reason why crudité platters, soup or salad should be reserved for company.

fats, fats, fats

By now you've probably heard that fat isn't all bad, right? You know that you should be increasing your intake of healthy fats like olive oil, canola oil, nut oils, and eating avocados and fatty fish like salmon and sardines regularly. Your body needs good fat to operate correctly: your brain, immune system and nervous system especially.

New research is showing that low-fat diets are more detrimental than diets that include healthy fats. Why? Because people began eating more sugar, simple carbohydrates and reduced-fat, processed meats such as ham or deli-style turkey.

But, before you run out and buy a stick of butter, consider the case for plant-based fats. In many cases they have been shown to *improve* your health, while butter has only been shown not to *harm* your health. So, while moderate use of butter won't do you any harm, moderate use of plant-based oils like the ones listed above, will actually benefit your health.

How in the world are we mere humans supposed to keep track of what's good and what's bad? Reports of research suggest first one approach, and then later, sometimes a month or several years later, it suggests something completely different. Focusing on real, plant-based food is the best guideline.

When using olive, avocado or nut oils, buy first expeller, cold pressed so that the nutrients have been preserved. It's also best to buy them in a size that allows you to use it up in a reasonable amount of time otherwise you take the risk of it becoming rancid. Check online or contact the manufacturer to find out the smoke point of your favorite cooking oil and use that as a guide for how to use it. Heating an oil past its smoke point will cause the release of free radicals. According to the Mayo Clinic, corn, peanut, soybean and sesame oils can handle high heats, while canola and olive oil are good for medium heat such as sautéing[xvii]. (I recommend sourcing your fats from non-GMO plants.)

In looking at the studies quoted and misquoted, once again what comes to the fore is your best choice is to follow a diet similar to a traditional Mediterranean Diet: lots and lots of fruits and vegetables, whole grains, mostly plant-based healthy fats, whether saturated or not, small amounts of animal products, high quality yogurt and cheese, and definitely fish.

The bottom line: Quit focusing on *low* fat and focus on adding in healthy fats.

learn to cook at home

WHY? You need to be in control of the quality of ingredients that go into your body and the bodies of your family. Most restaurants' goals are that the food they serve tastes good and is cheap to produce (even in the fancy, expensive restaurants). What they're not concerned with are the health effects of heavy cream and cheap oils. Remember, you are what you eat ... quite literally!

I know it takes time, but if you develop a plan to spend a few hours researching recipes online, preparing a general plan and a grocery list, adding the time into your calendar and following through, you'll be set for the week! (Note: When you find a recipe that sounds good online, read the comments left by people who have tried the recipes and you'll learn what worked, what didn't, what substitutions or additions were successful and you will probably get the advice you need that will make it more to your liking.)

There are several good recipe websites which allow you to save your recipes, but I like using Evernote for that. It's an application that you can have on your computer, tablet and smartphone which allows you to have the ingredients at your fingertips while shopping and cooking. Evernote allows you to save the web page as a 'simplified article' which eliminates all or most of the advertising.

If you're not an online kinda person, check out cookbooks from your library. You won't get the comments (which I find invaluable) but you'll have a never-ending supply of recipes.

New to cooking? Start simple! You don't want to try a complicated recipe the first time out. You might even consider starting with a cookbook designed for children. I love the family cooking magazine, *ChopChop*! It was the recipient of a James Beard award, includes interesting interviews, and has a focus on food diversity and health. It is recommended by 50% of the nation's pediatricians! True, it's designed for children, but I've made recipes from it and recommend it to clients who want simple, tasty and healthy ideas.

Okay, trust me, you can follow a recipe. Just gather the measuring equipment, pots, pans and ingredients, and commit to reading each step carefully. Then cook one new meal a week until you have a list of favorites. That will allow you time to get used to the process, time to fail and succeed and definitely time to learn what you like and don't like.

A quick note: By cook, I don't mean open up a bag of frozen dinner mix, toss in some chicken and call it homemade. What I do mean is learn to cook meals from scratch. As food manufacturers provide more and more pre-assembled meals, scratch cooking is becoming extinct, and with it so is our health. Also, most restaurants and take-outs use ingredients that are less costly and are heavy handed with a salt shaker, butter and cream. That Tomato Bisque soup isn't deliciously creamy because they know something you don't, it's because they use something you don't: heavy cream.

reduce sodium increase potassium*

You're probably sick to death of people telling you to reduce your salt intake, but how often do you hear them advise you to increase potassium? We all know that excess sodium can cause issues with high blood pressure, but did you know that getting sufficient potassium from whole foods can reduce blood pressure?

What's the best approach to achieve a healthy balance between sodium and potassium? Choose whole, real food, significantly reduce processed foods, and when you do use salt, choose the natural variety. Humans need salt; we just need to get it in more natural forms. I like Celtic Sea and Himalayan salts (Cooking at home improves the quality of our food drastically!)

The great thing about the combination is that when you increase potassium intake you automatically decrease sodium intake. Why? Your overall plan is to eat more whole foods, and that's exactly where you'll find potassium. In most cases, whole foods are very low in sodium! Here is a list of whole foods, fresh or frozen, that are high in potassium:

- avocados
- dried apricots

- raisins
- beans/peas
- soybeans/tofu
- mushrooms
- bananas
- greens, spinach, kale
- oranges and grapefruit
- melons
- sardines
- tuna
- peanuts
- walnuts
- sweet potatoes
- tomatoes

Why is it important to get your potassium from whole foods? You don't run the risk of overdoing it. There is an intricate balancing act that occurs between sodium and potassium, and as we age our kidneys don't excrete potassium as efficiently as they once did. That's not a problem when you fulfill your requirements with food.

*Some medical conditions require careful monitoring of potassium. As always, if you have a medical condition or are taking prescription drugs, check with your physician before changing your diet.

try fermented bread

Another reason we're seeing a higher incidence of gluten intolerances is that prior to the 1950's bread was made using a natural, long fermentation process during which enzymes, acting on the gluten, broke it down into amino acids that our body recognized and could use as building blocks at the cellular level. What this means today is that if you're sensitive to gluten, and you can find a company or baker that uses a fermentation time of 12+ hours you will probably be able to eat their bread without issue.

Even if you don't choose to eliminate gluten, you can benefit from the wholesomeness of this tasty bread. I live near a local bakery that makes a delicious fermented, sprouted rye that I find irresistible!

There is a lot of talk about people with Celiac being able to eat properly fermented sourdough, often citing a small Italian study that followed six participants. If I had Celiac Disease I'm not sure I'd be the first in line at the bakery. There is more research underway studying the effects of fermentation on wheat, but for someone with Celiac, it is better to be safe and wait for results.

the vending
machine is calling

How is it that a machine can call to you? You know it does! Two o'clock comes around and all of a sudden you're hearing that sweet, mechanical voice whispering to you from down the hall. What's it saying exactly? It's either sweet or salty, maybe both?

I used to hear the call of Snickers® but it was occasionally interrupted by that of Cheetos®. I don't work in an office building anymore, but in our culture, gas stations and drug stores are worse than vending machines. They are vending machines on steroids!

My clients and I have found a new superpower! When we hear the call it just doesn't have the same impact as it once did. Why? We travel with healthy snacks. Try storing dried fruit and nuts in your desk drawer and have a handful of peanuts and mini-boxes of raisins in your car at all times. Many of my clients have had their biggest success with this single tip.

Why does this work? Sugar, fat. protein and fiber. Rather than loading up on fake food, your body responds to the combination of natural sugar that enters your system slowly because the fat, protein and fiber slow it down. What does that mean for you? Sustained energy, no hunger, and goodbye to answering the call!

So, fix yourself some vending machine-repellant packages and have them with you at all times—in your desk, your car and/or your purse, because in today's world things are stressful enough without the constant temptation of junk food taking us down.

Claim your superpower!

sugar

I am simply not going to go into all of the statistics about how much sugar is in soda or candy bars or even ketchup. Instead, I'm going to recommend that you go back to the sections *Be Good to Your Gut, Read Labels, Who Controls Your Taste Buds, Kick Soda to the Curb, Go Ahead ... Try a Detox, Be Good to Your Heart, Curb Cravings, Relapse Prevention and Portion Control* ... WHEW! That should tell you something about the power of sugar!

One of the most powerful things you can do for your health is to eliminate sugar. This is true whether or not you're genetically predisposed to diabetes. I cannot tell you how much better you will feel. That doesn't mean you should add artificial sweeteners into your diet; just get all of that excess sweetness gone!

As I said in the section on detoxing, the cravings decrease quite quickly when you cut sugar out of your diet completely. But not all sugars are created equal, and that's the good news. You can enjoy fresh fruit, frozen fruit and even canned fruit if it's packed in 100% fruit juice and you discard the juice. (Fruit juices have as much or more sugar than sweetened sodas so don't turn to them as an alternative.)

Eat an apple or an orange, squeeze orange juice into a glass of seltzer but please, please, please lose the sugar!

so, this is it!

We've gone through many choices, so pick one that resonates with where you're at right now. Some people have had good luck by picking one or two of the easier choices first so they had a taste of success right away. Others are more motivated by a challenge, so they go all out and choose one that's much harder.

If you're interested in general health you can focus on anything you wish, but if your doctor has advised you to change your diet in ways that will have an impact on a chronic condition, then focus on making changes that will support your specific health concerns.

I'm going out on a limb here, but I don't believe you can be healthy without addressing the following five things.

- Healthy Eating
- Movement
- Healthy Environment
- Sleep
- Hydration

If you eat healthy but don't move, your body and brain will eventually revolt and cause a multitude of health problems. If you eat healthy, hydrate and have fun, but don't sleep well, you aren't giving your body and brain time to regenerate.

You can see where I'm going here. Your health, the health of both your body and your mind are contingent upon your attention to each of those categories. Whether you are 20 or 70, you are significantly impacting your health with each simple change you add in.

This series isn't designed to be a quick fix. It's designed to be used as a lifelong guide to how you can effect change in your life. I work with this concept whenever I need to get a handle on a lifestyle challenge, and I hope it works as well for you as it does for me.

If you have children, using the tracking sheets is a great way to get them on board as well. Remember, adding in one healthy habit at a time adds up to big rewards!

The next book in the series will address the other categories of building a healthy lifestyle, but for now let's get started on those eating habits.

Go out and get healthy!

I absolutely love speaking to organizations, companies, schools, gyms, community centers and health fairs. Please check out the programs I currently offer and feel free to contact via email at:
info@healthworkskc.com

Remember to have fun! Thinking of change as positive, and an adventure, will make all the difference in the world!

let's track it!

My Simple Change	M	T	W	R	F	S	S

Remember to have fun! Thinking of change as positive, and an adventure, will make all the difference in the world!

let's track it!

My Simple Change	M	T	W	R	F	S	S

bibliography

[i] Antioxidants: Beyond the Hype. (2016). Retrieved November 17, 2016, from
https://www.hsph.harvard.edu/nutritionsource/antioxidants/

[ii] 2 Knapton, S. (n.d.). Swap statins for a daily apple to improve heart health, say health experts. Retrieved November 17, 2016, from
http://www.telegraph.co.uk/news/health/news/12115433/Swap-statins-for-a-daily-apple-to-improve-heart-health-say-health-experts.html

[iii] What's New and Beneficial About Apples. (n.d.). Retrieved August 7, 2016, from
http://www.whfoods.com/genpage.php?tname=foodspice&dbid=15

[iv] Khanna, S., MBBS, MS, & Tosh, P. K., MD. (2014, January). A Clinician's Primer on the Role of the Microbiome in ... Retrieved November 19, 2016, from
http://www.mayoclinicproceedings.org/article/S0025-6196(13)00886-0/pdf

[v] Weil, A., MD. (n.d.). Love Me, Love My Microbiome - Dr. Andrew Weil. Retrieved July/August, 2016, from
http://www.drweil.com/health-wellness/body-mind-spirit/gastrointestinal/love-me-love-my-microbiome/

[vi] Bittman, M. (2012, July 24). More on Milk. Retrieved July/August, 2016, from
http://opinionator.blogs.nytimes.com/2012/07/24/more-on-milk/

[vii] Bittman, M. (2012, July 7). Got Milk? You Don't Need It. Retrieved August, 2012, from
http://opinionator.blogs.nytimes.com/2012/07/07/got-milk-you-dont-need-it/

viii Christensen, J. (2015, June 16). FDA on trans-fat: Halt use in U.S. food within 3 years. Retrieved July/August, 2016, from http://www.cnn.com/2015/06/16/health/fda-trans-fat/index.html

ix Trans Fats. (2015, October 7). Retrieved July/August, 2016, from http://www.heart.org/HEARTORG/HealthyLiving/HealthyEating/Nutrition/Trans-Fats_UCM_301120_Article.jsp

x Myers, A., MD. (2013, January 22). 10 Signs You're Gluten Intolerant. Retrieved July/August, 2016, from http://www.mindbodygreen.com/0-7482/10-signs-youre-gluten-intolerant.html

xi Ujjawal, K. (2016). *Black Rice Research, History and Development* (Illustrated ed., Vol. 1). Springer. Retrieved July/August, 2016, Pg. 154

xii Seeds, chia seeds, dried Nutrition Facts & Calories. (n.d.). Retrieved August/September, 2016, from http://nutritiondata.self.com/facts/nut-and-seed-products/3061/2

xiii Lussier, N. (n.d.). CHIAPIOCA: CHIA SEED PUDDING. Retrieved from http://realfoodswitch.com/tag/chia-seed-pudding/

xiv MyPlate Daily Checklist. (2016, January). Retrieved August/September, 2016, from https://choosemyplate-prod.azureedge.net/sites/default/files/myplate/checklists/MyPlateDailyChecklist_2000cals_Age14plus.pdf

xv McDonald's Nutrition Calculator | McDonald's. (n.d.). Retrieved September, 2016, from https://www.mcdonalds.com/us/en-us/about-our-food/nutrition-calculator.html

xvi Nutrition Calculator. (n.d.). Retrieved September, 2016, from https://www.tacobell.com/food/nutrition/calculator

xvii Zeratsky, K., RD, LD. (n.d.). Which type of oil should I use for cooking with high heat? Retrieved August/September, 2016, from http://www.mayoclinic.org/healthy-lifestyle/nutrition-and-healthy-eating/expert-answers/cooking-oil/faq-20058170

www.ingramcontent.com/pod-product-compliance
Lightning Source LLC
Chambersburg PA
CBHW050544280326
41933CB00011B/1717